As a Matter of Course

by Annie Payson

PREFACE.

THE aim of this book is to assist towards the removal of nervous irritants, which are not only the cause of much physical disease, but materially interfere with the best possibilities of usefulness and pleasure in everyday life.

CONTENTS.

AS A MATTER OF COURSE.

I.

INTRODUCTION.

IN climbing a mountain, if we know the path and take it as a matter of course, we are free to enjoy the beauties of the surrounding country. If in the same journey we set a stone in the way and recognize our ability to step over it, we do so at once, and save ourselves from tripping or from useless waste of time and thought as to how we might best go round it.

There are stones upon stones in every-day life which might be stepped over with perfect ease, but which, curiously enough, are considered from all sides and then tripped upon; and the result is a stubbing of the moral toes, and a consequent irritation of the nervous system. Or, if semi-occasionally one of these stones is stepped over as a matter of course, the danger is that attention is immediately called to the action by admiring friends, or by the person himself, in a way so to tickle the nervous system that it amounts to an irritation, and causes him to trip over the next stone, and finally tumble on his nose. Then, if he is not wise enough to pick himself up and walk on with the renewed ability of stepping over future stones, he remains on his nose far longer than is either necessary or advisable.

These various stones in the way do more towards keeping a nervous system in a chronic state of irritation than is imagined. They are what might perhaps be called the outside elements of life. These once normally faced, cease to exist as impediments, dwindle away, and finally disappear altogether.

Thus we are enabled to get nearer the kernel, and have a growing realization of life itself.

Civilization may give a man new freedom, a freedom beyond any power of description or conception, except to those who achieve it, or it may so bind him body and soul that in moments when he recognizes his nervous contractions he would willingly sell his hope of immortality to be a wild horse or tiger for the rest of his days.

These stones in the way are the result of a perversion of civilization, and the cause of much contraction and unnecessary suffering.

There is the physical stone. If the health of the body were attended to as a matter of course, as its cleanliness is attended to by those of us who are more civilized, how much easier life might be! Indeed, the various trippings on, and endeavors to encircle, this physical stone, raise many phantom stones, and the severity of the fall is just as great when one trips over a stone that is not there. Don Quixote was quite exhausted when he had been fighting the windmills. One recognizes over and over the truth spoken by the little girl who, when reprimanded by her father for being fretful, said: "It isn't me, papa, it's that banana."

There is also the over-serious stone; and this, so far from being stepped over or any effort made to encircle it, is often raised to the undue dignity of a throne, and not rested upon. It seems to produce an inability for any sort of recreation, and a scorn of the necessity or the pleasure of being amused. Every one will admit that recreation is one swing of life's pendulum; and in proportion to the swing in that direction will be the strength of the swing in the other direction, and vice versa.

One kind of stone which is not the least among the self-made impediments is the microscopic faculty which most of us possess for increasing small, inoffensive pebbles to good-sized rocks. A quiet insistence on seeing these pebbles in their natural size would reduce them shortly to a pile of sand which might be easily smoothed to a level, and add to the comfort of the path. Moods are stones which not only may be stepped over, but kicked right out of the path with a good bold stroke. And the stones of intolerance may be replaced by an open sympathy,--an ability to take the other's point of view,--which will bring flowers in the path instead.

In dealing with ourselves and others there are stones innumerable, if one chooses to regard them, and a steadily decreasing number as one steps over and ignores. In our relations with illness and poverty, so-called, the ghosts of stones multiply themselves as the illness or the poverty is allowed to be a limit rather than a guide. And there is nothing that exorcises all such ghosts more truly than a free and open intercourse with little children.

If we take this business of slipping over our various nerve-stones as a matter of course, and not as a matter of sentiment, we get a powerful result just as surely as we get powerful results in obedience to any other practical laws.

In bygone generations men used to fight and kill one another for the most trivial cause. As civilization increased, self-control was magnified into a virtue, and the man who governed himself and allowed his neighbor to escape unslain was regarded as a hero. Subsequently, general slashing was found to be incompatible with a well-ordered community, and forbearance in killing or scratching or any other unseemly manner of attacking an enemy was taken as a matter of course.

Nowadays we do not know how often this old desire to kill is repressed, a brain-impression of hatred thereby intensified, and a nervous irritation caused which has its effect upon the entire disposition. It would hardly be feasible to return to the killing to save the irritation that follows repression; civilization has taken us too far for that. But civilization does not necessarily mean repression. There are many refinements of barbarity in our civilization which might be dropped now, as the coarser expressions of such states were dropped by our ancestors to enable them to reach the present stage of knives and forks and napkins. And inasmuch as we are farther on the way towards a true civilization, our progress should be more rapid than that of our barbaric grandfathers. An increasingly accelerated progress has proved possible in scientific research and discovery; why not, then, in our practical dealings with ourselves and one another?

Does it not seem likely that the various forms of nervous irritation, excitement, or disease may result as much from the repressed savage within us as from the complexity of civilization? The remedy is, not to let the savage have his own way; with many of us, indeed, this would be difficult, because of the generations of repression behind us. It is to cast his skin, so to speak, and rise to another order of living.

Certainly repression is only apparent progress. No good physician would allow it in bodily disease, and, on careful observation, the law seems to hold good in other phases of life.

There must be a practical way by which these stones, these survivals of barbaric times, may be stepped over and made finally to disappear.

The first necessity is to take the practical way, and not the sentimental. Thus true sentiment is found, not lost.

The second is to follow daily, even hourly, the process of stepping over until it comes to be indeed a matter of course. So, little by little, shall we emerge from this mass of abnormal nervous irritation into what is more truly life itself.
II.

PHYSICAL CARE.

REST, fresh air, exercise, and nourishment, enough of each in proportion to the work done, are the material essentials to a healthy physique. Indeed, so simple is the whole process of physical care, it would seem absurd to write about it at all. The only excuse for such writing is the constant disobedience to natural laws which has resulted from the useless complexity of our civilization.

There is a current of physical order which, if one once gets into it, gives an instinct as to what to do and what to leave undone, as true as the instinct which leads a man to wash his hands when they need it, and to wash them often enough so that they never remain soiled for any length of time, simply because that state is uncomfortable to their owner. Soap and water are not unpleasant to most of us in their process of cleansing; we have to deny ourselves nothing through their use. To keep the digestion in order, it is often necessary to deny ourselves certain sensations of the palate which are pleasant at the time. So by a gradual process of not denying we are swung out of the instinctive nourishment-current, and life is complicated for us either by an amount of thought as to what we should or should not eat, or by irritations which arise from having eaten the wrong food. It is not uncommon to find a mind taken up for some hours in wondering whether that last piece of cake will digest. We can easily see how from this there might be developed a nervous sensitiveness about eating which would prevent the individual from eating even the food that is nourishing. This last is a not unusual form of dyspepsia,--a dyspepsia which keeps itself alive on the patient's want of nourishment.

Fortunately the process of getting back into the true food-current is not difficult if one will adopt it The trouble is in making the bold plunge. If anything is eaten that is afterwards deemed to have been imprudent, let it disagree. Take the full consequences and bear them like a man, with whatever remedies are found to lighten the painful result. Having made sure through bitter experience that a particular food disagrees, simply do not take it again, and think nothing about it. It does not exist for you. A nervous resistance to any sort of indigestion prolongs the attack and leaves, a brain-impression which not only makes the same trouble more liable to recur, but increases the temptation to eat forbidden fruit. Of course this is always preceded by a full persuasion that the food is not likely to disagree with us now simply because it did before. And to some extent, this is true. Food that will bring pain and suffering when taken by a tired stomach, may prove entirely nourishing when the stomach is rested and ready for it. In that case, the owner of the stomach has learned once for all never to give his digestive apparatus work to do when it is tired. Send a warm drink as a messenger to say that food is coming later, give yourself a little rest, and then eat your dinner. The fundamental laws of health in eating are very simple; their variations for individual needs must be discovered by each for himself.

"But," it may be objected, "why make all this fuss, why take so much thought about what I eat or what I do not eat?" The special thought is simply to be taken at first to get into the normal habit, and as a means of forgetting our digestion just as we forget the washing of our hands until we are reminded by some discomfort; whereupon we wash them and forget again.

Nature will not allow us to forget. When we are not obeying her laws, she is constantly irritating us in one way or another. It is when we obey, and obey as a matter of course, that she shows herself to be a tender mother, and helps us to a real companionship with her.

Nothing is more amusing, nothing could appeal more to Mother Nature's sense of humor, than the various devices for exercise which give us a complicated self-consciousness rather than a natural development of our physical powers. Certain simple exercises are most useful, and if the weather is so inclement that they cannot be taken in the open air, it is good to have a well-ventilated hall. Exercise with others, too, is stimulating, and more invigorating when there is air enough and to spare. But there is nothing that shows the subjective, self-conscious state of this generation more than the subjective form which exercise takes. Instead of games and play or a good vigorous walk in the country, there are endless varieties of physical culture, most of it good and helpful if taken as a means to an end, but almost useless as it is taken as an end in itself; for it draws the attention to one's self and one's own muscles in a way to make the owner serve the muscle instead of the muscle being made to serve the owner. The more physical exercise can be simplified and made objective, the more it serves its end. To climb a high mountain is admirable exercise, for we have the summit as an end, and the work of climbing is steadily objective, while we get the delicious effect of a freer circulation and all that it means. There might be similar exercises in gymnasiums, and there are, indeed, many exercises where some objective achievement is the end, and the training of a muscle follows as a matter of course. There is the exercise-instinct; we all have it the more perfectly as we obey it. If we have suffered from a series of disobediences, it is a comparatively easy process to work back into obedience.

The fresh-air-instinct is abnormally developed with some of us, but only with some. The popular fear of draughts is one cause of its loss. The fear of a draught will cause a contraction, the contraction will interfere with the circulation, and a cold is the natural result.

The effect of vitiated air is well known. The necessity, not only for breathing fresh air when we are quiet, but for exercising in the open, grows upon us as we see the result. To feel the need is to take the remedy, as a matter of course.

The rest-instinct is most generally disobeyed, most widely needed, and obedience to it would bring the most effective results. A restful state of mind and body prepares one for the best effects from exercise, fresh air, and nourishment. This instinct is the more disobeyed because with the need for rest there seems to come an inability to take it, so that not only is every impediment magnified, but imaginary impediments are erected, and only a decided and insistent use of the will in dropping everything that interferes, whether real or imaginary, will bring a whiff of a breeze from the true rest-current. Rest is not always silence, but silence is always rest; and a real silence of the mind is known by very few. Having gained that, or even approached it, we are taken by the rest-wind itself, and it is strong enough to bear our full weight as it swings us along to renewed life and new strength for work to come.

The secret is to turn to silence at the first hint from nature; and sleep should be the very essence of silence itself.

All this would be very well if we were free to take the right amount of rest, fresh air, exercise, and nourishment; but many of us are not. It will not be difficult for any one to call to mind half a dozen persons who impede the good which might result from the use of these four necessities simply by complaining that they cannot have their full share of either. Indeed, some of us may find in ourselves various stones of this sort stopping the way. To take what we can and be thankful, not only enables us to gain more from every source of health, but opens the way for us to see clearly how to get more. This complaint, however, is less of an impediment than the whining and fussing which come from those who are free to take all four in abundance, and who have the necessity of their own especial physical health so much at heart that there is room to think of little else. These people crowd into the various schools of physical culture by the hundred, pervade the rest-cures, and are ready for any new physiological fad which may arise, with no result but more physical culture, more rest-cure, and more fads. Nay, there is sometimes one other result,--disease. That gives them something tangible to work for or to work about. But all their eating and breathing and exercising and resting does not bring lasting vigorous health, simply because they work at it as an end, of which self is the centre and circumference.

The sooner our health-instinct is developed, and then taken as a matter of course, the sooner can the body become a perfect servant, to be treated with true courtesy, and then forgotten. Here is an instinct of our barbarous ancestry which may be kept and refined through all future phases of civilization. This instinct is natural, and the obedience to it enables us to gain more rapidly in other, higher instincts which, if our ancestors had at all, were so embryonic as not to have attained expression.

Nourishment, fresh air, exercise, rest,--so far as these are not taken simply and in obedience to the natural instinct, there arise physical stones in the way, stones that form themselves into an apparently insurmountable wall. There is a stile over that wall, however, if we will but open our eyes to see it. This stile, carefully climbed, will enable us to step over the few stones on the other side, and follow the physical path quite clearly.

III.

AMUSEMENTS.

THE ability to be easily and heartily amused brings a wholesome reaction from intense thought or hard work of any kind which does more towards keeping the nervous system in a normal state than almost anything else of an external kind.

As a Frenchman very aptly said: "This is all very well, all this study and care to relieve one's nerves; but would it not be much simpler and more effective to go and amuse one's self ?" The same Frenchman could not realize that in many countries amusement is almost a lost art. Fortunately, it is not entirely lost; and the sooner it is regained, the nearer we shall be to health and happiness.

One of the chief impediments in the way of hearty amusement is over-seriousness. There should be two words for "serious," as there are literally two meanings. There is a certain intense form of taking the care and responsibility of one's own individual interests, or the interests of others which are selfishly made one's own, which leads to a surface-seriousness that is not only a chronic irritation of the nervous system, but a constant distress to those who come under this serious care. This is taking life au grand serieux.

The superficiality of this attitude is striking, and would be surprising could the sufferer from such seriousness once see himself (or more often it is herself) in a clear light. It is quite common to call such a person over-serious, when in reality he is not serious enough. He or she is laboring under a sham seriousness, as an actor might who had such a part to play and merged himself in the character. These people are simply exaggerating their own importance to life, instead of recognizing life's importance to them. An example of this is the heroine of Mrs. Ward's "Robert Elsmere," who refused to marry because the family could not get on without her; and when finally she consented, the family lived more happily and comfortably than when she considered herself their leader. If this woman's seriousness, which blinded her judgment, had been real instead of sham, the state of the case would have been quite clear to her; but then, indeed, there would have been no case at all.

When seriousness is real, it is never intrusive and can never be overdone. It is simply a quiet, steady obedience to recognized laws followed as a matter of course, which must lead to a clearer appreciation of such laws, and of our own freedom in obeying them. Whereas with a sham seriousness we dwell upon the importance of our own relation to the law, and our own responsibility in forcing others to obey. With the real, it is the law first, and then my obedience. With the sham, it is myself first, and then the laws; and often a strained obedience to laws of my own making.

This sham seriousness, which is peculiarly a New England trait, but may also be found in many other parts of the world, is often the perversion of a strong, fine nature. It places many stones in the way, most of them phantoms, which, once stepped over and then ignored, brings to light a nature nobly expansive, and a source of joy to all who come in contact with it. But so long as the "seriousness "lasts, it is quite incompatible with any form of real amusement.

For the very essence of amusement is the child-spirit. The child throws himself heartily and spontaneously into the game, or whatever it may be, and forgets that there is anything else in the world, for the time being. Children have nothing else to remember. We have the advantage of them there, in the pleasure of forgetting and in the renewed strength with which we can return to our work or care, in consequence. Any one who cannot play children's games with children, and with the same enjoyment that children have, does not know the spirit of amusement. For this same spirit must be taken into all forms of amusement, especially those that are beyond the childish mind, to bring the delicious reaction which nature is ever ready to bestow. This is almost a self-evident truth; and yet so confirmed is man in his sham maturity that it is quite common to see one look with contempt, and a sense of superiority which is ludicrous, upon another who is enjoying a child's game like a child. The trouble is that many of us are so contracted in and oppressed by our own self-consciousness that open spontaneity is out of the question and even inconceivable. The sooner we shake it off, the better. When the great philosopher said, "Except ye become as little children," he must have meant it all the way through in spirit, if not in the letter. It certainly is the common-sense view, whichever way we look at it, and proves as practical as walking upon one's feet.

With the spontaneity grows the ability to be amused, and with that ability comes new power for better and really serious work.

To endeavor with all your might to win, and then if you fail, not to care, relieves a game of an immense amount of unnecessary nervous strain. A spirit of rivalry has so taken hold of us and become such a large stone in the way, that it takes wellnigh a reversal of all our ideas to realize that this same spirit is quite compatible with a good healthy willingness that the other man should win--if he can. Not from the goody-goody motive of wishing your neighbor to beat,--no neighbor would thank you for playing with him in that spirit,--but from a feeling that you have gone in to beat, you have done your best, as far as you could see, and where you have not, you have learned to do better. The fact of beating is not of paramount importance. Every man should have his chance, and, from your opponent's point of view, provided you were as severe on him as you knew how to be at the time, it is well that he won. You will see that it does not happen again.

Curious it is that the very men or women who would scorn to play a child's game in a childlike spirit, will show the best known form of childish fretfulness and sheer naughtiness in their way of taking a game which is considered to be more on a level with the adult mind, and so rasp their nerves and the nerves of their opponents that recreation is simply out of the question.

Whilst one should certainly have the ability to enjoy a child's game with a child and like a child, that not only does not exclude the preference which many, perhaps most of us may have for more mature games, it gives the power to play those games with a freedom and ease which help to preserve a healthy nervous system.

If, however, amusement is taken for the sole purpose of preserving a normal nervous system, or for returning to health, it loses its zest just in proportion. If, as is often the case, one must force one's self to it at first, the love of the fun will gradually come as one ignores the first necessity of forcing; and the interest will come sooner if a form of amusement is taken quite opposite to the daily work, a form which will bring new faculties and muscles into action.

There is, of course, nothing that results in a more unpleasant state of ennui than an excess of amusement. After a certain amount of careless enjoyment, life comes to a deadly stupid standstill, or the forms of amusement grow lower. In either case the effect upon the nervous system is worse even than over-work.

The variety in sources of amusement is endless, and the ability to get amusement out of almost anything is delightful, as long as it is well balanced.

After all, our amusement depends upon the way in which we take our work, and our work, again, depends upon the amusement; they play back and forth into one another's hands.

The man or the woman who cannot get the holiday spirit, who cannot enjoy pure fun for the sake of fun, who cannot be at one with a little child, not only is missing much in life that is clear happiness, but is draining his nervous system, and losing his better power for work accordingly.

This anti-amusement stone once removed, the path before us is entirely new and refreshing.

The power to be amused runs in nations. But each individual is in himself a nation, and can govern himself as such; and if he has any desire for the prosperity of his own kingdom, let him order a public holiday at regular intervals, and see that the people enjoy it.

IV.

BRAIN IMPRESSIONS.

THE mere idea of a brain clear from false impressions gives a sense of freedom which is refreshing.

In a comic journal, some years ago, there was a picture of a man in a most self-important attitude, with two common mortals in the background gazing at him. "What makes him stand like that?" said one. "Because," answered the other, "that is his own idea of himself." The truth suggested in that picture strikes one aghast; for in looking about us we see constant examples of attitudinizing in one's own idea of one's self. There is sometimes a feeling of fright as to whether I am not quite as abnormal in my idea of myself as are those about me.

If one could only get the relief of acknowledging ignorance of one's self, light would be welcome, however given. In seeing the truth of an unkind criticism one could forget to resent the spirit; and what an amount of nerve-friction might be saved! Imagine the surprise of a man who, in return for a volley of abuse, should receive thanks for light thrown upon a false attitude. Whatever we are enabled to see, relieves us of one mistaken brain-impression, which we can replace by something more agreeable. And if, in the excitement of feeling, the mistake was exaggerated, what is that to us? All we wanted was to see it in quality. As to degree, that lessens in proportion as the quality is bettered. Fortunately, in living our own idea of ourselves, it is only ourselves we deceive, with possible exceptions in the case of friends who are so used to us, or so over-fond of us, as to lose the perspective.

There is the idea of humility,--an obstinate belief that we know we are nothing at all, and deserve no credit; which, literally translated, means we know we are everything, and deserve every credit. There is the idea, too, of immense dignity, of freedom from all self-seeking and from all vanity. But it is idle to attempt to catalogue these various forms of private theatricals; they are constantly to be seen about us.

It is with surprise unbounded that one hears another calmly assert that he is so-and-so or so-and-so, and in his next action, or next hundred actions, sees that same assertion entirely contradicted. Daily familiarity with the manifestations of mistaken brain- impressions does not lessen one's surprise at this curious personal contradiction; it gives one an increasing desire to look to one's self, and see how far these private theatricals extend in one's own case, and to throw off the disguise, as far as it is seen, with a full acknowledgment that there may be--probably is--an abundance more of which to rid one's self in future. There are many ways in which true openness in life, one with another, would be of immense service; and not the least of these is the ability gained to erase false brain-impressions.

The self-condemnatory brain-impression is quite as pernicious as its opposite. Singularly enough, it goes with it. One often finds inordinate self-esteem combined with the most abject condemnation of self. One can be played against the other as a counter-irritant; but this only as a process of rousing, for the irritation of either brings equal misery. I am not even sure that as a rousing process it is ever really useful. To be clear of a mistaken brain-impression, a man must recognize it himself; and this recognition can never be brought about by an unasked attempt of help from another. It is often cleared by help asked and given; and perhaps more often by help which is quite involuntary and unconscious. One of the greatest points in friendly diplomacy is to be open and absolutely frank so far as we are asked, but never to go beyond. At least, in the experience of many, that leads more surely to the point where no diplomacy is needed, which is certainly the point to be aimed at in friendship. It is trying to see a friend living his own idea of himself, and to be obliged to wait until he has discovered that he is only playing a part. But this very waiting may be of immense assistance in reducing our own moral attitudinizing.

How often do we hear others or find ourselves complaining of a fault over and over again! "I know that is a fault of mine, and has been for years. I wish I could get over it." "I know that is a fault of mine,"--one brain-impression; "it has been for years,"--a dozen or more brain-impressions, according to the number of years; until we have drilled the impression of that fault in, by emphasizing it over and over, to an extent which daily increases the difficulty of dropping it.

So, if we have the habit of unpunctuality, and emphasize it by deploring it, it keeps us always behind time. If we are sharp-tongued, and dwell with remorse on something said in the past, it increases the tendency in the future.

The slavery to nerve habit is a well-known physiological fact; but nerve habit may be strengthened negatively as well as positively. When this is more widely recognized, and the negative practice avoided, much will have been done towards freeing us from our subservience to mistaken brain-impressions.

Let us take an instance: unpunctuality-for example, as that is a common form of repetition. If we really want to rid ourselves of the habit, suppose every time we are late we cease to deplore it; make a vivid mental picture of ourselves as being on time at the next appointment; then, with the how and the when clearly impressed upon our minds, there should be an absolute refusal to imagine ourselves anything but early. Surely that would be quite as effective as a constant repetition of the regret we feel at being late, whether this is repeated aloud to others, or only in our own minds. As we place the two processes side by side, the latter certainly has the advantage, and might be tried, until a better is found.

Of course we must beware of getting an impression of promptness which has no ground in reality. It is quite possible for an individual to be habitually and exasperatingly late, with all the air and innocence of unusual punctuality.

It would strike us as absurd to see a man painting a house the color he did not like, and go on painting it the same color, to show others and himself that which he detested. Is it not equally absurd for any of us, through the constant expression of regret for a fault, to impress the tendency to it more and more upon the brain? It is intensely sad when the consciousness of evil once committed has so impressed a man with a sense of guilt as to make him steadily undervalue himself and his own powers.

Here is a case where one's own idea of one's self is seventy-five per cent below par; and a gentle and consistent encouragement in raising that idea is most necessary before par is reached

And par, as I understand it, is simple freedom from any fixed idea of one's self, either good or bad.

If fixed impressions of one's self are stones in the way, the same certainly holds good with fixed impressions of others. Unpleasant brain-impressions of others are great weights, and greater impediments in the way of clearing our own brains. Suppose So- and-so had such a fault yesterday; it does not follow that he has not rid himself of at least part of it to-day. Why should we hold the brain-impression of his mistake, so that every time we look at him we make it stronger? He is not the gainer thereby, and we certainly are the losers. Repeated brain-impressions of another's faults prevent our discerning his virtues. We are constantly attributing to him disagreeable motives, which arise solely from our idea of him, and of which he is quite innocent. Not only so, but our mistaken impressions increase his difficulty in rising to the best of himself. For any one whose temperament is in the least sensitive is oppressed by what he feels to be another's idea of him, until he learns to clear himself of that as well as of other brain-impressions.

It is not uncommon to hear one go over and over a supposed injury, or even small annoyances from others, with the reiterated assertion that he fervently desires to forget such injury or annoyances. This fervent desire to forgive and forget expresses itself by a repeated brain-impression of that which is to be forgiven; and if this is so often repeated in words, how many times more must it be repeated mentally! Thus, the brain-impression is increased until at last forgetting seems out of the question. And forgiving is impossible unless one can at the same time so entirely forget the ill-feeling roused as to place it beyond recall.

Surely, if we realized the force and influence of unpleasant brain-impressions, it would be a simple matter to relax and let them escape, to be replaced by others that are only pleasant It cannot be that we enjoy the discomfort of the disagreeable impressions.

And yet, so curiously perverted is human nature that we often hear a revolting story told with the preface, "Oh, I can't bear to think of it! "And the whole story is given, with a careful attention to detail which is quite unnecessary, even if there were any reason for telling the story at all, and generally concluded with a repetition of the prefatory exclamation. How many pathetic sights are told of, to no end but the repetition of an unpleasant brain-impression. How many past experiences, past illnesses, are gone over and over, which serve the same worse than useless purpose,--that of repeating and emphasizing the brain-impression.

A little pain is made a big one by persistent dwelling upon it; what might have been a short pain is sometimes lengthened for a lifetime. Similarly, an old pain is brought back by recalling a brain-impression.

The law of association is well known. We all know how familiar places and happenings will recall old feelings; we can realize this at any time by mentally reviving the association. By dwelling on the pain we had yesterday we are encouraging it to return to-morrow. By emphasizing the impression of an annoyance of to-day we are making it possible to suffer beyond expression from annoyances to come; and the annoyances, the pains, the disagreeable feelings will find their old brain-grooves with remarkable rapidity when given the ghost of a chance.

I have known more than one case where a woman kept herself ill by the constant repetition, to others and to herself, of a nervous shock. A woman who had once been frightened by burglars refused to sleep for fear of being awakened by more burglars, thus increasing her impression of fear; and of course, if she slept at all, she was liable at any time to wake with a nervous start. The process of working herself into nervous prostration through this constant, useless repetition was not slow.

The fixed impressions of preconceived ideas in any direction are strangely in the way of real freedom. It is difficult to catch new harmonies with old ones ringing in our ears; still more difficult when we persist in listening at the same time to discords.

The experience of arguing with another whose preconceived idea is so firmly fixed that the argument is nothing but a series of circles, might be funny if it were not sad; and it often is funny, in spite of the sadness.

Suppose we should insist upon retaining an unpleasant brain-impression, only when and so long as it seemed necessary in order to bring a remedy. That accomplished, suppose we dropped it on the instant. Suppose, further, that we should continue this process, and never allow ourselves to repeat a disagreeable brain-impression aloud or mentally. Imagine the result. Nature abhors a vacuum; something must come in place of the unpleasantness; therefore way is made for feelings more comfortable to one's self and to others.

Bad feelings cause contraction, good ones expansion. Relax the muscular contraction; take a long, free breath of fresh air, and expansion follows as a matter of course. Drop the brain-contraction, take a good inhalation of whatever pleasant feeling is nearest, and the expansion is a necessary consequence.

As we expand mentally, disagreeable brain-impressions, that in former contracted states were eclipsed by greater ones, will be keenly felt, and dropped at once, for the mere relief thus obtained.

The healthier the brain, the more sensitive it is to false impressions, and the more easily are they dropped.

One word by way of warning. We never can rid ourselves of an uncomfortable brain-impression by saying, "I will try to think something pleasant of that disagreeable man." The temptation, too, is very common to say to ourselves clearly, "I will try to think something pleasant," and then leave "of that disagreeable man" a subtle feeling in the background. The feeling in the background, however unconscious we may be of it, is a strong brain-impression,--all the stronger because we fail to recognize it,--and the result of our "something pleasant" is an insidious complacency at our own magnanimous disposition. Thus we get the disagreeable brain-impression of another, backed up by our agreeable brain-impression of ourselves, both mistaken. Unless we keep a sharp look-out, we may here get into a snarl from which extrication is slow work. Neither is it possible to counteract an unpleasant brain-impression by something pleasant but false. We must call a spade a spade, but not consider it a component part of the man who handles it, nor yet associate the man with the spade, or the spade with the man. When we drop it, so long as we drop it for what it is worth, which is nothing in the case of the spade in question, we have dropped it entirely. If we try to improve our brain-impression by insisting that a spade is something better and pleasanter, we are transforming a disagreeable impression to a mongrel state which again brings anything but a happy result.

Simply to refuse all unpleasant brain-impressions, with no effort or desire to recast them into something that they are not, seems to be the only clear process to freedom. Not only so, but whatever there might have been pleasant in what seemed entirely unpleasant can more truly return as we drop the unpleasantness completely. It is a good thing that most of us can approach the freedom of such a change in imagination before we reach it in reality. So we can learn more rapidly not to hamper ourselves or others by retaining disagreeable brain-impressions of the present, or by recalling others of the past.

V.

THE TRIVIALITY OF TRIVIALITIES.

LIFE is clearer, happier, and easier for us as things assume their true proportions. I might better say, as they come nearer in appearance to their true proportions; for it seems doubtful whether any one ever reaches the place in this world where the sense of proportion is absolutely normal. Some come much nearer than others; and part of the interest of living is the growing realization of better proportion, and the relief from the abnormal state in which circumstances seem quite out of proportion in their relation to one another.

Imagine a landscape-painter who made his cows as large as the houses, his blades of grass waving above the tops of the trees, and all things similarly disproportionate. Or, worse, imagine a disease of the retina which caused a like curious change in the landscape itself wherein a mountain appeared to be a mole-hill, and a mole-hill a mountain.

It seems absurd to think of. And, yet, is not the want of a true sense of proportion in the circumstances and relations of life quite as extreme with many of us? It is well that our physical sense remains intact. If we lost that too, there would seem to be but little hope indeed. Now, almost the only thing needed for a rapid approach to a more normal mental sense of proportion is a keener recognition of the want. But this want must be found first in ourselves, not in others. There is the inclination to regard our own life as bigger and more important than the life of any one about us; or the reverse attitude of bewailing its lack of importance, which is quite the same.

In either case our own life is dwelt upon first. Then there is the immediate family, after that our own especial friends,--all assuming a gigantic size which puts quite out of the question an occasional bird's-eye view of the world in general. Even objects which might be in the middle distance of a less extended view are quite screened by the exaggerated size of those which seem to concern us most immediately.

One's own life is important; one's own family and friends are important, very, when taken in their true proportion. One should surely be able to look upon one's own brothers and sisters as if they were the brothers and sisters of another, and to regard the brothers and sisters of another as one's own. Singularly, too, real appreciation of and sympathy with one's own grows with this broader sense of relationship. In no way is this sense shown more clearly than by a mother who has the breadth and the strength to look upon her own children as if they belonged to some one else, and upon the children of others as if they belonged to her. But the triviality of magnifying one's own out of all proportion has not yet been recognized by many.

So every trivial happening in our own lives or the lives of those connected with us is exaggerated, and we keep ourselves and others in a chronic state of contraction accordingly.

Think of the many trifles which, by being magnified and kept in the foreground, obstruct the way to all possible sight or appreciation of things that really hold a more important place. The cook, the waitress, various other annoyances of housekeeping; a gown that does not suit, the annoyances of travel, whether we said the right thing to so-and-so, whether so-and-so likes us or does not like us,--indeed, there is an immense army of trivial imps, and the breadth of capacity for entertaining these imps is so large in some of us as to be truly encouraging; for if the domain were once deserted by the imps, there remains the breadth, which must have the same capacity for holding something better. Unfortunately, a long occupancy by these miserable little offenders means eventually the saddest sort of contraction. What a picture for a new Gulliver!--a human being overwhelmed by the imps of triviality, and bound fast to the ground by manifold windings of their cobweb-sized thread.

This exaggeration of trifles is one form of nervous disease. It would be exceedingly interesting and profitable to study the various phases of nervous disease as exaggerated expressions of perverted character. They can be traced directly and easily in many cases. If a woman fusses about trivialities, she fusses more when she is tired. The more fatigue, the more fussing; and with a persistent tendency to fatigue and fussing it does not take long to work up or down to nervous prostration. From this form of nervous excitement one never really recovers, except by a hearty acknowledgment of the trivialities as trivialities, when, with growing health, there is a growing sense of true proportion.

I have seen a woman spend more attention, time, and nerve-power on emphasizing the fact that her hands were all stained from the dye on her dress than a normal woman would take for a good hour's work. As she grew better, this emphasizing of trivialities decreased, but, of course, might have returned with any over-fatigue, unless it had been recognized, taken at its worth, and simply dropped. Any one can think of example after example in his own individual experience, when he has suffered unnecessary tortures through the regarding of trifling things, either by himself or by some one near him. With many, the first instance will probably be to insist, with emphasis and some feeling, that they are not trivialities.

Trivialities have their importance when given their true proportion. The size of a triviality is often exaggerated as much by neglect as by an undue amount of attention. When we do what we can to amend an annoyance, and then think no more about it until there appears something further to do, the saving of nervous force is very great. Yet, so successful have these imps of triviality come to be in their rule of human nature that the trivialities of the past are oftentimes dwelt upon with as much earnestness as if they belonged to the present.

The past itself is a triviality, except in its results. Yet what an immense screen it is sometimes to any clear understanding or appreciation of the present! How many of us have listened over and over to the same tale of past annoyances, until we wonder how it can be possible that the constant repetition is not recognized by the narrator! How many of us have been over and over in our minds past troubles, little and big, so that we have no right whatever to feel impatient when listening to such repetitions by others! Here again we have, in nervous disease, the extreme of a common trait in humanity. With increased nervous fatigue there is always an increase of the tendency to repetition. Best drop it before it gets to the fatigue stage, if possible.

Then again there are the common things of life, such as dressing and undressing, and the numberless every-day duties. It is possible to distort them to perfect monstrosities by the manner of dwelling upon them. Taken as a matter of course, they are the very triviality of trivialities, and assume their place without second thought.

When life seems to get into such a snarl that we despair of disentangling it, a long journey and change of human surroundings enable us to take a distant view, which not uncommonly shows the tangle to be no tangle at all. Although we cannot always go upon a material journey, we can change the mental perspective, and it is this adjustment of the focus which brings our perspective into truer proportions. Having once found what appears to be the true focus, let us be true to it. The temptations to lose one's focus are many, and sometimes severe. When temporarily thrown off our balance, the best help is to return at once, without dwelling on the fact that we have lost the focus longer than is necessary to find it again. After that, our focus is better adjusted and the range steadily expanded. It is impossible for us to widen the range by thinking about it; holding the best focus we know in our daily experience does that Thus the proportions arrange themselves; we cannot arrange the proportions. Or, what is more nearly the truth, the proportions are in reality true, to begin with. As with the imaginary eye-disease, which transformed the relative sizes of the component parts of a landscape, the fault is in the eye, not in the landscape; so, when the circumstances of life are quite in the wrong proportion to one another, in our own minds, the trouble is in the mental sight, not in the circumstances.

There are many ways of getting a better focus, and ridding one's self of trivial annoyances. One is, to be quiet; get at a good mental distance. Be sure that you have a clear view, and then hold it. Always keep your distance; never return to the old stand-point if you can manage to keep away.

We may be thankful if trivialities annoy us as trivialities. It is with those who have the constant habit of dwelling on them without feeling the discomfort that a return to freedom seems impossible.

As one comes to realize, even in a slight degree, the triviality of trivialities, and then forget them entirely in a better idea of true proportion, the sense of freedom gained is well worth working for. It certainly brings the possibility of a normal nervous system much nearer.

VI.

MOODS.

RELIEF from the mastery of an evil mood is like fresh air after having been several hours in a close room.

If one should go to work deliberately to break up another's nervous system, and if one were perfectly free in methods of procedure, the best way would be to throw upon the victim in rapid sequence a long series of the most extreme moods. The disastrous result could be hastened by insisting that each mood should be resisted as it manifested itself, for then there would be the double strain,--the strain of the mood, and the strain of resistance. It is better to let a mood have its way than to suppress it. The story of the man who suffered from varicose veins and was cured by the waters of Lourdes, only to die a little later from an affection of the heart which arose from the suppression of the former disease, is a good illustration of the effect of mood-suppression. In the case cited, death followed at once; but death from repeated impressions of moods resisted is long drawn out, and the suffering intense, both for the patient and for his friends.

The only way to drop a mood is to look it in the face and call it by its right name; then by persistent ignoring, sometimes in one way, sometimes in another, finally drop it altogether. It takes a looser hold next time, and eventually slides off entirely. To be sure, over-fatigue, an attack of indigestion, or some unexpected contact with the same phase in another, may bring back the ghost of former moods. These ghosts may even materialize, unless the practice of ignoring is at once referred to; but they can ultimately be routed completely.

A great help in gaining freedom from moods is to realize clearly their superficiality. Moods are deadly, desperately serious things when taken seriously and indulged in to the full extent of their power. They are like a tiny spot directly in front of the eye. We see that, and that only. It blurs and shuts out everything else. We groan and suffer and are unhappy and wretched, still persistently keeping our eye on the spot, until finally we forget that there is anything else in the world. In mind and body we are impressed by that and that alone. Thus the difficulty of moving off a little distance is greatly increased, and liberation is impossible until we do move away, and, by a change of perspective, see the spot for what it really is.

Let any one who is ruled by moods, in a moment when he is absolutely free from them, take a good look at all past moody states, and he will see that they come from nothing, go to nothing, and, are nothing. Indeed, that has been and is often done by the moody person, with at the same time an unhappy realization that when the moods are on him, they are as real as they are unreal when he is free. To treat a mood as a good joke when you are in its clutches, is simply out of the question. But to say, "This now is a mood. Come on, do your worst; I can stand it as long as you can," takes away all nerve-resistance, until the thing has nothing to clutch, and dissolves for want of nourishment. If it proves too much for one at times, and breaks out in a bad expression of some sort, a quick acknowledgment that you are under the spell of a bad mood, and a further invitation to come on if it wants to, will loosen the hold again.

If the mood is a melancholy one, speak as little as possible under its influence; go on and do whatever there is to be done, not resisting it in any way, but keep busy.

This non-resistance can, perhaps, be better illustrated by taking, instead of a mood, a person who teases. It is well known that the more we are annoyed, the more our opponent teases; and that the surest and quickest way of freeing ourselves is not to be teased. We can ignore the teaser externally with an internal irritation which he sees as clearly as if we expressed it. We can laugh in such a way that every sound of our own voice proclaims the annoyance we are trying to hide. It is when we take his words for what they are worth, and go with him, that the wind is taken out of his sails, and he stops because there is no fun in it. The experience with a mood is quite parallel, though rather more difficult at first, for there is no enemy like the enemies in one's self, no teasing like the teasing from one's self. It takes a little longer, a little heartier and more persistent process of non-resistance to cure the teasing from one's own nature. But the process is just as certain, and the freedom greater in result.

Why is it not clear to us that to set our teeth, clench our hands, or hold any form of extreme tension and mistaken control, doubles, trebles, quadruples the impression of the feeling controlled, and increases by many degrees its power for attacking us another time? Persistent control of this kind gives a certain sort of strength. It might be called sham strength, for it takes it out of one in other ways. But the control that comes from non-resistance brings a natural strength, which not only steadily increases, but spreads on all sides, as the growth of a tree is even in its development.

"If a man takes your cloak, give him your coat also; if one compel you to go a mile, go with him twain." "Love your enemies, do good to them that hurt you, and pray for them that despitefully use you." Why have we been so long in realizing the practical, I might say the physiological, truth of this great philosophy? Possibly because in forgiving our enemies we have been so impressed with the idea that it was our enemies we were forgiving. If we realized that following this philosophy would bring us real freedom, it would be followed steadily as a matter of course, and with no more sense that we deserved credit for doing a good thing than a man might have in walking out of prison when his jailer opened the door. So it is with our enemies the moods.

I have written heretofore of bad moods only. But there are moods and moods. In a degree, certainly, one should respect one's moods. Those who are subject to bad moods are equally subject to good ones, and the superficiality of the happier modes is just as much to be recognized as that of the wretched ones. In fact, in recognizing the shallowness of our happy moods, we are storing ammunition for a healthy openness and freedom from the opposite forms. With the full realization that a mood is a mood, we can respect it, and so gradually reach a truer evenness of life. Moods are phases that we are all subject to whilst in the process of finding our balance; the more sensitive and finer the temperament, the more moods. The rhythm of moods is most interesting, and there is a spice about the change which we need to give relish to these first steps towards the art of living.

It is when their seriousness is exaggerated that they lose their power for good and make slaves of us. The seriousness may be equally exaggerated in succumbing to them and in resisting them. In either case they are our masters, and not our slaves. They are steady consumers of the nervous system in their ups and downs when they master us; and of course retain no jot of that fascination which is a good part of their very shallowness, and brings new life as we take them as a matter of course. Then we are swung in their rhythm, never once losing sight of the point that it is the mood that is to serve us, and not we the mood.

As we gain freedom from our own moods, we are enabled to respect those of others and give up any endeavor to force a friend out of his moods, or even to lead him out, unless he shows a desire to be led. Nor do we rejoice fully in the extreme of his happy moods, knowing the certain reaction.

Respect for the moods of others is necessary to a perfect freedom from our own. In one sense no man is alone in the world; in another sense every man is alone; and with moods especially, a man must be left to work out his own salvation, unless he asks for help. So, as he understands his moods, and frees himself from their mastery, he will find that moods are in reality one of Nature's gifts, a sort of melody which strengthens the harmony of life and gives it fuller tone.

Freedom from moods does not mean the loss of them, any more than non-resistance means allowing them to master you. It is non-resistance, with the full recognition of what they are, that clears the way.

VII.

TOLERANCE.

WHEN we are tolerant as a matter of course, the nervous system is relieved of almost the worst form of persistent irritation it could have.

The freedom of tolerance can only be appreciated by those who have known the suffering of intolerance and gained relief.

A certain perspective is necessary to a recognition of the full absurdity of intolerance. One of the greatest absurdities of it is evident when we are annoyed and caused intense suffering by our intolerance of others, and, as a consequence, blame others for the fatigue or illness which follows. However mistaken or blind other people may be in their habits or their ideas, it is entirely our fault if we are annoyed by them. The slightest blame given to another in such a case, on account of our suffering, is quite out of place.

Our intolerance is often unconscious. It is disguised under one form of annoyance or another, but when looked full in the face, it can only be recognized as intolerance.

Of course, the most severe form is when the belief, the action, or habit of another interferes directly with our own selfish aims. That brings the double annoyance of being thwarted and of rousing more selfish antagonism.

Where our selfish desires are directly interfered with, or even where an action which we know to be entirely right is prevented, intolerance only makes matters worse. If expressed, it probably rouses bitter feelings in another. Whether we express it openly or not, it keeps us in a state of nervous irritation which is often most painful in its results. Such irritation, if not extreme in its effect, is strong enough to keep any amount of pure enjoyment out of life.

There may be some one who rouses our intolerant feelings, and who may have many good points which might give us real pleasure and profit; but they all go for nothing before our blind, restless intolerance.

It is often the case that this imaginary enemy is found to be a friend and ally in reality, if we once drop the wretched state of intolerance long enough to see him clearly.

Yet the promptest answer to such an assertion will probably be, "That may be so in some cases, but not with the man or woman who rouses my intolerance."

It is a powerful temptation, this one of intolerance, and takes hold of strong natures; it frequently rouses tremendous tempests before it can be recognized and ignored. And with the tempest comes an obstinate refusal to call it by its right name, and a resentment towards others for rousing in us what should not have been there to be roused.

So long as a tendency to anything evil is in us, it is a good thing to have it roused, recognized, and shaken off; and we might as reasonably blame a rock, over which we stumble, for the bruises received, as blame the person who rouses our intolerance for the suffering we endure.

This intolerance, which is so useless, seems strangely absurd when it is roused through some interference with our own plans; but it is stranger when we are rampant against a belief which does not in any way interfere with us.

This last form is more prevalent in antagonistic religious beliefs than in anything else. The excuse given would be an earnest desire for the salvation of our opponent. But who ever saved a soul through an ungracious intolerance of that soul's chosen way of believing or living? The danger of loss would seem to be all on the other side.

One's sense of humor is touched, in spite of one's self, to hear a war of words and feeling between two Christians whose belief is supposed to be founded on the axiom, "Judge not, that ye be not judged."

Without this intolerance, argument is interesting, and often profitable. With it, the disputants gain each a more obstinate belief in his own doctrines; and the excitement is steadily destructive to the best health of the nervous system.

Again, there is the intolerance felt from various little ways and habits of others,--habits which are comparatively nothing in themselves, but which are monstrous in their effect upon a person who is intolerant of them.

One might almost think we enjoyed irritated nerves, so persistently do we dwell upon the personal peculiarities of others. Indeed, there is no better example of biting off one's own nose than the habit of intolerance. It might more truly be called the habit of irritating one's own nervous system.

Having recognized intolerance as intolerance, having estimated it at its true worth, the next question is, how to get rid of it. The habit has, not infrequently, made such a strong brain-impression that, in spite of an earnest desire to shake it off, it persistently clings.

Of course, the soil about the obnoxious growth is loosened the moment we recognize its true quality. That is a beginning, and the rest is easier than might be imagined by those who have not tried it.

Intolerance is an unwillingness that others should live in their own way, believe as they prefer to, hold personal habits which they enjoy or are unconscious of, or interfere in any degree with our ways, beliefs, or habits.

That very sense of unwillingness causes a contraction of the nerves which is wasteful and disagreeable. The feeling rouses the contraction, the contraction more feeling; and so the Intolerance is increased in cause and in effect. The immediate effect of being willing, on the contrary, is, of course, the relaxation of such contraction, and a healthy expansion of the nerves.

Try the experiment on some small pet form of intolerance. Try to realize what it is to feel quite willing. Say over and over to yourself that you are quite willing So-and-so should make that curious noise with his mouth. Do not hesitate at the simplicity of saying the words to yourself; that brings a much quicker effect at first. By and by we get accustomed to the sensation of willingness, and can recall it with less repetition of words, or without words at all. When the feeling of nervous annoyance is roused by the other, counteract it on the instant by repeating silently: "I am quite willing you should do that,--do it again." The man or woman, whoever he or she may be, is quite certain to oblige you! There will be any number of opportunities to be willing, until by and by the willingness is a matter of course, and it would not be surprising if the habit passed entirely unnoticed, as far as you are concerned.

This experiment tried successfully on small things can be carried to greater. If steadily persisted in, a good fifty per cent of wasted nervous force can be saved for better things; and this saving of nervous force is the least gain which comes from a thorough riddance of every form of intolerance.

"But," it will be objected, "how can I say I am willing when I am not?"

Surely you can see no good from the irritation of unwillingness; there can be no real gain from it, and there is every reason for giving it up. A clear realization of the necessity for willingness, both for our own comfort and for that of others, helps us to its repetition in words. The words said with sincere purpose, help us to the feeling, and so we come steadily into clearer light.

Our very willingness that a friend should go the wrong way, if he chooses, gives us new power to help him towards the right. If we are moved by intolerance, that is selfishness; with it will come the desire to force our friend into the way which we consider right. Such forcing, if even apparently successful, invariably produces a reaction on the friend's part, and disappointment and chagrin on our own.

The fact that most great reformers were and are actuated by the very spirit of intolerance, makes that scorning of the ways of others seem to us essential as the root of all great reform. Amidst the necessity for and strength in the reform, the petty spirit of intolerance intrudes unnoticed. But if any one wants to see it in full-fledged power, let him study the family of a reformer who have inherited the intolerance of his nature without the work to which it was applied.

This intolerant spirit is not indispensable to great reforms; but it sometimes goes with them, and is made use of, as intense selfishness may often be used, for higher ends. The ends might have been accomplished more rapidly and more effectually with less selfish instruments. But man must be left free, and if he will not offer himself as an open channel to his highest impulses, he is used to the best advantage possible without them.

There is no finer type of a great reformer than Jesus Christ; in his life there was no shadow of intolerance. From first to last, he showed willingness in spirit and in action. In upbraiding the Scribes and Pharisees he evinced no feeling of antagonism; he merely stated the facts. The same firm calm truth of assertion, carried out in action, characterized his expulsion of the money-changers from the temple. When he was arrested, and throughout his trial and execution, it was his accusers who showed the intolerance; they sent out with swords and staves to take him, with a show of antagonism which failed to affect him in the slightest degree.

Who cannot see that, with the irritated feeling of intolerance, we put ourselves on the plane of the very habit or action we are so vigorously condemning? We are inviting greater mistakes on our part. For often the rouser of our selfish antagonism is quite blind to his deficiencies, and unless he is broader in his way than we are in ours, any show of intolerance simply blinds him the more. Intolerance, through its indulgence, has come to assume a monstrous form. It interferes with all pleasure in life; it makes clear, open intercourse with others impossible; it interferes with any form of use into which it is permitted to intrude. In its indulgence it is a monstrosity,--in itself it is mean, petty, and absurd.

Let us then work with all possible rapidity to relax from contractions of unwillingness, and become tolerant as a matter of course.

Whatever is the plan of creation, we cannot improve it through any antagonistic feeling of our own against creatures or circumstances. Through a quiet, gentle tolerance we leave ourselves free to be carried by the laws. Truth is greater than we are, and if we can be the means of righting any wrong, it is by giving up the presumption that we can carry truth, and by standing free and ready to let truth carry us.

The same willingness that is practised in relation to persons will be found equally effective in relation to the circumstances of life, from the losing of a train to matters far greater and more important. There is as much intolerance to be dropped in our relations to various happenings as in our relations to persons; and the relief to our nerves is just as great, perhaps even greater.

It seems to be clear that heretofore we have not realized either the relief or the strength of an entire willingness that people and things should progress in their own way. How can we ever gain freedom whilst we are entangled in the contractions of intolerance?

Freedom and a healthy nervous system are synonymous; we cannot have one without the other.

VIII.

SYMPATHY.

SYMPATHY, in its best sense, is the ability to take another's point of view. Not to mourn because he mourns; not to feel injured because he feels injured. There are times when we cannot agree with a friend in the necessity for mourning or feeling injured; but we can understand the cause of his disturbance, and see clearly that his suffering is quite reasonable, from his own point of view. One cannot blame a man for being color-blind; but by thoroughly understanding and sympathizing with the fact that red must be green as he sees it, one can help him to bring his mental retina to a more normal state, until every color is taken at its proper value.

This broader sort of sympathy enables us to serve others much more truly.

If we feel at one with a man who is suffering from a supposed injury which may be entirely his own fault, we are doing all in our power to confirm him in his mistake, and his impression of martyrdom is increased and protracted in proportion. But if, with a genuine comprehension of his point of view, however unreal it may be in itself, we do our best to see his trouble in an unprejudiced light, that is sympathy indeed; for our real sympathy is with the man himself, cleared from his selfish fog. What is called our sympathy with his point of view is more a matter of understanding. The sympathy which takes the man for all in all, and includes the comprehension of his prejudices, will enable us to hold our tongues with regard to his prejudiced view until he sees for himself or comes to us for advice.

It is interesting to notice how this sympathy with another enables us to understand and forgive one from whom we have received an injury. His point of view taken, his animosity against us seems to follow as a matter of course; then no time or force need be wasted on resentment.

Again, you cannot blame a man for being blind, even though his blindness may be absolutely and entirely selfish, and you the sufferer in consequence.

It often follows that the endeavor to get a clear understanding of another's view brings to notice many mistaken ideas of our own, and thus enables us to gain a better standpoint It certainly helps us to enduring patience; whereas a positive refusal to regard the prejudices of another is rasping to our own nerves, and helps to fix him in whatever contraction may have possessed him.

There can be no doubt that this open sympathy is one of the better phases of our human intercourse most to be desired. It requires a clear head and a warm heart to understand the prejudices of a friend or an enemy, and to sympathize with his capabilities enough to help him to clearer mental vision.

Often, to be sure, there are two points of view, both equally true. But they generally converge into one, and that one is more easily found through not disputing our own with another's. Through sympathy with him we are enabled to see the right on both sides, and reach the central point.

It is singular that it takes us so long to recognize this breadth of sympathy and practise it. Its practice would relieve us of an immense amount of unnecessary nerve-strain. But the nerve-relief is the mere beginning of gain to come. It steadily opens a clearer knowledge and a heartier appreciation of human nature. We see in individuals traits of character, good and bad, that we never could have recognized whilst blinded by our own personal prejudices. By becoming alive to various little sensitive spots in others, we are enabled to avoid them, and save an endless amount of petty suffering which might increase to suffering that was really severe.

One good illustration of this want of sympathy, in a small way, is the waiting-room of a well-known nerve-doctor. The room is in such a state of confusion, it is such a mixture of colors and forms, that it would be fatiguing even for a person in tolerable health to stay there for an hour. Yet the doctor keeps his sensitive, nervously excited patients sitting in this heterogeneous mass of discordant objects hour after hour. Surely it is no psychological subtlety of insight that gives a man of this type his name and fame: it must be the feeding and resting process alone; for a man of sensitive sympathy would study to save his patients by taking their point of view, as well as to bring them to a better physical state through nourishment and rest

The ability to take a nervous sufferer's point of view is greatly needed. There can be no doubt that with that effort on the part of friends and relatives, many cases of severe nervous prostration might be saved, certainly much nervous suffering could be prevented.

A woman who is suffering from a nervous conscience writes a note which shows that she is worrying over this or that supposed mistake, or as to what your attitude is towards her. A prompt, kind, and direct answer will save her at once from further nervous suffering of that sort. To keep an anxious person, whether he be sick or well, watching the mails, is a want of sympathy which is also shown in many other ways, unimportant, perhaps, to us, but important if we are broad enough to take the other's point of view.

There are many foolish little troubles from which men and women suffer that come only from tired nerves. A wise patience with such anxieties will help greatly towards removing their cause. A wise patience is not indulgence. An elaborate nervous letter of great length is better answered by a short but very kind note.

The sympathy which enables us to understand the point of view of tired nerves gives us the power to be lovingly brief in our response to them, and at the same time more satisfying than if we responded at length.

Most of us take human nature as a great whole, and judge individuals from our idea in general. Or, worse, we judge it all from our own personal prejudices. There is a grossness about this which we wonder at not having seen before, when we compare the finer sensitiveness which is surely developed by the steady effort to understand another's point of view. We know a whole more perfectly as a whole if we have a distinct knowledge of the component parts. We can only understand human nature en masse through a daily clearer knowledge of and sympathy with its individuals. Every one of us knows the happiness of having at least one friend whom he is perfectly sure will neither undervalue him nor give him undeserved praise, and whose friendship and help he can count upon, no matter how great a wrong he has done, as securely as he could count upon his loving thought and attention in physical illness. Surely it is possible for each of us to approach such friendship in our feeling and attitude towards every one who comes in touch with us.

It is comparatively easy to think of this open sympathy, or even practise it in big ways; it is in the little matters of everyday life that the difficulty arises. Of course the big ways count for less if they come through a brain clogged with little prejudices, although to some extent one must help the other.

It cannot be that a man has a real open sympathy who limits it to his own family and friends; indeed, the very limit would make the open sympathy impossible. One is just as far from a clear comprehension of human nature when he limits himself by his prejudices for his immediate relatives as when he makes himself alone the boundary.

Once having gained even the beginning of this broader sympathy with others, there follows the pleasure of freedom from antagonisms, keener delight in understanding others, individually and collectively, and greater ability to serve others; and all these must give an impetus which takes us steadily on to greater freedom, to clearer understanding, and to more power to serve and to be served.

Others have many experiences which we have never even touched upon. In that case, our ability to understand is necessarily limited. The only thing to do is to acknowledge that we cannot see the point of view, that we have no experience to start from, and to wait with an open mind until we are able to understand.

Curiously enough, it is precisely these persons of limited experience who are most prone to prejudice. I have heard a man assert with emphasis that it was every one's duty to be happy, who had apparently not a single thing in life to interfere with his own happiness. The duty may be clear enough, but he certainly was not in a position to recognize its difficulty. And just in proportion with his inability to take another's point of view in such difficulty did he miss his power to lead others to this agreeable duty.

There are, of course, innumerable things, little and big, which we shall be enabled to give to others and to receive from others as the true sympathy grows.

The common-sense of it all appeals to us forcibly.

Who wants to carry about a mass of personal prejudices when he can replace them by the warm, healthy feeling of sympathetic friendship? Who wants his nerves to be steadily irritated by various forms of intolerance when, by understanding the other's point of view, he can replace these by better forms of patience?

This lower relief is little compared with the higher power gained, but it is the first step up, and the steps beyond go ever upward. Human nature is worth knowing and worth loving, and it can never be known or loved without open sympathy.

Why, we ourselves are human nature!

Many of us would be glad to give sympathy to others, especially in little ways, but we do not know how to go to work about it; we seem always to be doing the wrong thing, when our desire is to do the right. This comes, of course, from the same inability to take the other's point of view; and the ability is gained as we are quiet and watch for it.

Practice, here as in everything else, is what helps. And the object is well worth working for.

IX.

OTHERS.

HOW to live at peace with others is a problem which, if practically solved, would relieve the nervous system of a great weight, and give to living a lightness and ease that might for a time seem weirdly unnatural. It would certainly decrease the income of the nerve-specialists to the extent of depriving those gentlemen of many luxuries they now enjoy.

Peace does not mean an outside civility with an inside dislike or annoyance. In that case, the repressed antagonism not only increases the brain-impression and wears upon the nervous system, but it is sure to manifest itself some time, in one form or another; and the longer it is repressed, the worse will be the effect. It may be a volcanic eruption that is produced after long repression, which simmers down to a chronic interior grumble; or it may be that the repression has caused such steadily increasing contraction that an eruption is impossible. In this case, life grows heavier and heavier, burdened with the shackles of one's own dislikes.

If we can only recognize two truths in our relations with others, and let these truths become to us a matter of course, the worst difficulties are removed. Indeed, with these two simple bits of rationality well in hand, we may safely expect to walk amicably side by side with our dearest foe.

The first is, that dislike, nine times out often, is simply a "cutaneous disorder." That is, it is merely an irritation excited by the friction of one nervous system upon another. The tiny tempests in the tiny teapots which are caused by this nervous friction, the great weight attached to the most trivial matters of dispute, would touch one's sense of humor keenly if it were not that in so many cases these tiny tempests develop into real hurricanes. Take, for example, two dear and intimate friends who have lived happily together for years. Neither has a disposition which is perfect; but that fact has never interfered with their friendship. Both get over-tired. Words are spoken which sound intensely disagreeable, even cruel. They really express nothing in the world but tired nerves. They are received and misinterpreted by tired nerves on the other side. So these two sets of nerves act and react upon one another, and from nothing at all is evolved an ill-feeling which, if allowed to grow, separates the friends. Each is fully persuaded that his cutaneous trouble has profound depth. By a persistent refusal of all healing salves it sometimes sinks in until the disease becomes really deep seated. All this is so unnecessary. Through the same mistake many of us carry minor dislikes which, on account of their number and their very pettiness, are wearing upon the nerves, and keep us from our best in whatever direction we may be working.

The remedy for all these seems very clear when once we find it. Recognize the shallow-ness of the disorder, acknowledge that it is a mere matter of nerves, and avoid the friction. Keep your distance. It is perfectly possible and very comfortable to keep your distance from the irritating peculiarities of another, while having daily and familiar relations with him or her. The difficulty is in getting to a distance when we have allowed ourselves to be over-near; but that, too, can be accomplished with patience. And by keeping a nervous distance, so to speak, we are not only relieved from irritation, but we find a much more delightful friendship; we see and enjoy the qualities in another which the petty irritations had entirely obscured from our view. If we do not allow ourselves to be touched by the personal peculiarities, we get nearer the individual himself.

To give a simple example which would perhaps seem absurd if it had not been proved true so many times: A man was so annoyed by his friend's state of nervous excitability that in taking a regular morning walk with him, which he might have enjoyed heartily, he always returned fagged out He tried whilst walking beside his friend to put himself in imagination on the other side of the street The nervous irritation lessened, and finally ceased; the walk was delightful, and the friend--never suspected!

A Japanese crowd is so well-bred that no one person touches another; one need never jostle, but, with an occasional "I beg your pardon," can circulate with perfect ease. In such a crowd there can be no irritation.

There is a certain good-breeding which leads us to avoid friction with another's nervous system. It must, however, be an avoidance inside as well as outside. The subterfuge of holding one's tongue never works in the end. There is a subtle communication from one nervous system to another which is more insinuating than any verbal intercourse. Those nearest us, and whom we really love best, are often the very persons by whom we are most annoyed. As we learn to keep a courteous distance from their personal peculiarities our love grows stronger and more real; and an open frankness in our relation is more nearly possible. Strangely enough, too, the personal peculiarities sometimes disappear. It is possible, and quite as necessary, to treat one's own nervous system with this distant courtesy.

This brings us to the second simple truth. In nine cases out of ten the cause of this nervous irritation is in ourselves. If a man loses his temper and rouses us to a return attack, how can we blame him? Are we not quite as bad in hitting back? To be sure, he began it. But did he? How do we know what roused him? Then, too, he might have poured volleys of abuse upon us, and not provoked an angry retort, if the temper had not been latent within us, to begin with. So it is with minor matters. In direct proportion to our freedom from others is our power for appreciating their good points; just in proportion to our slavery to their tricks and their habits are we blinded to their good points and open to increased irritation from their bad ones. It is curious that it should work that way, but it does. If there is nothing in us to be roused, we are all free; if we are not free, it is because there is something in us akin to that which rouses us. This is hard to acknowledge. But it puts our attitude to others on a good clean basis, and brings us into reality and out of private theatricals; not to mention a clearing of the nervous system which gives us new power.

There is one trouble in dealing with people which does not affect all of us, but which causes enough pain and suffering to those who are under its influence to make up for the immunity of the rest. That is, the strong feeling that many of us have that it is our duty to reform those about us whose life and ways are not according to our ideas of right.

No one ever forced another to reform, against that other's will. It may have appeared so; but there is sure to be a reaction sooner or later. The number of nervous systems, however, that have been overwrought by this effort to turn others to better ways, is sad indeed. And in many instances the owners of these nervous systems will pose to themselves as martyrs; and they are quite sincere in such posing. They are living their own impressions of themselves, and wearing themselves out in consequence. If they really wanted right for the sake of right, they would do all in their power without intruding, would recognize the other as a free agent, and wait. But they want right because it is their way; consequently they are crushed by useless anxiety, and suffer superfluously. This is true of those who feel themselves under the necessity of reforming all who come in touch with them. It is more sadly true of those whose near friends seem steadily to be working out their own destruction. To stand aside and be patient in this last case requires strength indeed. But such patience clears one's mind to see, and gives power to act when action can prove effective. Indeed, as the ability to leave others free grows in us, our power really to serve increases.

The relief to the nervous system of dropping mistaken responsibility cannot be computed. For it is by means of the nervous system that we deal with others; it is the medium of our expression and of our impression. And as it is cleared of its false contractions, does it not seem probable that we might be opened to an exquisite delight in companionship that we never knew before, and that our appreciation of human nature would increase indefinitely?

Suppose when we find another whose ways are quite different from ours, we immediately contract, and draw away with the feeling that there is nothing in him for us. Or suppose, instead, that we look into his ways with real interest in having found a new phase of human nature. Which would be the more broadening process on the whole, or the more delightful?

Frequently the contraction takes more time and attention than would an effort to understand the strange ways. We are almost always sure to find something in others to which we can respond, and which awakens a new power in us, if only a new power of sympathy.

To sum it all up, the best way to deal with others seems to be to avoid nervous friction of any sort, inside or out; to harbor no ill-will towards another for selfishness roused in one's self; to be urged by no presumptive sense of responsibility; and to remember that we are all in the same world and under the same laws. A loving sympathy with human nature in general, leads us first to obey the laws ourselves, and gives us a fellow-feeling with individuals which means new strength on both sides.

To take this as a matter of course does not seem impossible. It is simply casting the skin of the savage and rising to another plane, where there will doubtless be new problems better worth attention.

X.

ONE'S SELF.

TO be truly at peace with one's self means rest indeed.

There is a quiet complacency, though, which passes for peace, and is like the remarkably clear red-and-white complexion which indicates disease. It will be noticed that the sufferers from this complacent spirit of so-called peace shrink from openness of any sort, from others or to others. They will put a disagreeable feeling out of sight with a rapidity which would seem to come from sheer fright lest they should see and acknowledge themselves in their true guise. Or they will acknowledge it to a certain extent, with a pleasure in their own humility which increases the complacency in proportion. This peace is not to be desired. With those who enjoy it, a true knowledge of or friendship with others is as much out of the question as a knowledge of themselves. And when it is broken or interfered with in any way, the pain is as intense and real as the peace was false.

The first step towards amicable relations with ourselves is to acknowledge that we are living with a stranger. Then it sometimes happens that through being annoyed by some one else we are enabled to recognize similar disagreeable tendencies in ourselves of which we were totally ignorant before.

As honest dealing with others always pays best in the end, so it is in all relations with one's self. There are many times when to be quite open with a friend we must wait to be asked. With ourselves no such courtesy is needed. We can speak out and done with it, and the franker we are, the sooner we are free. For, unlike other companions, we can enjoy ourselves best when we are conspicuous only by our own absence!

It is this constant persistence in clinging to ourselves that is most in the way; it increases that crown of nervous troubles, self-consciousness, and makes it quite impossible that we should ever really know ourselves. If by all this, we are not ineffable bores to ourselves, we certainly become so to other people.

It is surprising, when once we come to recognize it, how we are in an almost chronic state of posing to ourselves. Fortunately, a clear recognition of the fact is most effectual in stopping the poses. But they must be recognized, pose by pose, individually and separately stopped, and then ignored, if we want to free ourselves from ourselves entirely.

The interior posing-habit makes one a slave to brain-impressions which puts all freedom out of the question. To cease from such posing opens one of the most interesting gates to natural life. We wonder how we could have obscured the outside view for so long.

To find that we cannot, or do not, let ourselves alone for an hour in the day seems the more surprising when we remember that there is so much to enjoy outside. Egotism is immensely magnified in nervous disorders; but that it is the positive cause of much nervous trouble has not been generally admitted.

Let any one of us take a good look at the amount of attention given by ourselves to ourselves. Then acknowledge, without flinching, what amount of that attention is unnecessary; and it will clear the air delightfully, for a moment at any rate.

The tendency to refer everything, in some way or another, to one's self; the touchiness and suspicion aroused by nothing but petty jealousy as to one's own place; the imagined slights from others; the want of consideration given us,--all these and many more senseless irritations are in this over-attention to self. The worries about our own moral state take up so great a place with many of us as to leave no room for any other thought. Indeed, it is not uncommon to see a woman worrying so over her faults that she has no time to correct them. Self-condemnation is as great a vanity as its opposite. Either in one way or another there is the steady temptation to attend to one's self, and along with it an irritation of the nerves which keeps us from any sense of real freedom.

With most of us there is no great depth to the self-disease if it is only stopped in time. When once we are well started in the wholesome practice of getting rid of ourselves, the process is rapid. A thorough freedom from self once gained, we find ourselves quite companionable, which, though paradoxical, is without doubt a truth.

"That freedom of the soul," writes Fenelon, "which looks straight onward in its path, losing no time to reason upon its steps, to study them, or to dwell upon those already taken, is true simplicity." We recognize a mistake, correct it, go on and forget. If it appears again, correct it again. Irritation at the second or at any number of reappearances only increases the brain-impression of the mistake, and makes the tendency to future error greater.

If opportunity arises to do a good action, take advantage of it, and silently decline the disadvantage of having your attention riveted to it by the praise of others.

A man who is constantly analyzing his physical state is called a hypochondriac. What shall we call the man who is constantly analyzing his moral state? As the hypochondriac loses all sense of health in holding the impression of disease, so the other gradually loses the sense of wholesome relation to himself and to others.

If a man obeyed the laws of health as a matter of course, and turned back every time Nature convicted him of disobedience, he would never feel the need of self-analysis so far as his physical state was concerned. Just so far as a man obeys higher laws as a matter of course, and uses every mistake to enable him to know the laws better, is morbid introspection out of the question with him.

"Man, know thyself!" but, being sure of the desire to know thyself, do not be impatient at slow progress; pay little attention to the process, and forget thyself, except when remembering is necessary to a better forgetting.

To live at real peace with ourselves, we must surely let every little evil imp of selfishness show himself, and not have any skulking around corners. Recognize him for his full worthless-ness, call him by his right name, and move off. Having called him by his right name, our severity with ourselves for harboring him is unnecessary. To be gentle with ourselves is quite as important as to be gentle with others. Great nervous suffering is caused by this over-severity to one's self, and freedom is never accomplished by that means. Many of us are not severe enough, but very many are too severe. One mistake is quite as bad as the other, and as disastrous in its effects.

If we would regard our own state less, or careless whether we were happy or unhappy, our freedom from self would be gained more rapidly.

As a man intensely interested in some special work does not notice the weather, so we, if we once get hold of the immense interest there may be in living, are not moved to any depth by changes in the clouds of our personal state. We take our moods as a matter of course, and look beyond to interests that are greater. Self may be a great burden if we allow it. It is only a clear window through which we see and are seen, if we are free. And the repose of such freedom must be beyond our conception until we have found it. To be absolutely certain that we know ourselves at any time is one great impediment to reaching such rest. Every bit of self-knowledge gained makes us more doubtful as to knowledge to come. It would surprise most of us to see how really unimportant we are. As a part of the universe, our importance increases just in proportion to the laws that work through us; but this self-importance is lost to us entirely in our greater recognition of the laws. As we gain in the sensitive recognition of universal laws, every petty bit of self-contraction disappears as darkness before the rising of the sun.

XI.

CHILDREN.

WORK for the better progress of the human race is most effective when it is done through the children; for children are future generations. The freedom in mature life gained by a training that would enable the child to avoid nervous irritants is, of course, greatly in advance of most individual freedom to-day. This real freedom is the spirit of the kindergarten; but Frobel's method, as practised to-day, does not attack and put to rout all those various nervous irritants which are the enemies of our civilization. To be sure, the teaching of his philosophy develops such a nature that much pettiness is thrown off without even being noticed as a snare; and Frobel helps one to recognize all pettiness more rapidly. There are, however, many forms of nervous irritation which one is not warned against in the kindergarten, and the absence of which, if the child is taught as a matter of course to avoid them, will give him a freedom that his elders and betters (?) lack. The essential fact of this training is that it is only truly effectual when coming from example rather than precept.

A child is exquisitely sensitive to the shortcomings of others, and very keen, as well as correct, in his criticism, whether expressed or unexpressed. In so far as a man consents to be taught by children, does he not only remain young, but he frees himself from the habit of impeding his own progress. This is a great impediment, this unwillingness to be taught by those whom we consider more ignorant than ourselves because they have not been in the world so long. Did no one ever take into account the possibility of our eyes being blinded just because they had been exposed to the dust longer? Certainly one possible way of clearing this dust and avoiding it is to learn from observing those who have had less of it to contend with. Indeed, one might go so far as to say that no training of any child could be effectual to a lasting degree unless the education was mutual. When Frobel says, "Come, let us live with our children," he does not mean, Come, let us stoop to our children; he means, Let us be at one with them. Surely a more perfect harmony in these two great phases of human nature--the child and the man--would be greatly to the advantage of the latter.

Yet, to begin at the beginning, who ever feels the necessity of treating a baby with respect? How quickly the baby would resent intrusive attentions, if it knew how. Indeed, I have seen a baby not a year old resent being transferred from one person to another, with an expression of the face that was most eloquent. Women seem so full of their sense of possession of a baby that this eloquence is not even observed, and the poor child's nervous irritants begin at a very early age. There is so much to be gained by keeping at a respectful nervous distance from a baby, that one has only to be quiet enough to perceive the new pleasure once, to lose the temptation to interfere; and imagine the relief to the baby! It is, after all, the sense of possession that makes the trouble; and this sense is so strong that there are babies, all the way from twenty to forty, whose individuality is intruded upon so grossly that they have never known what freedom is; and when they venture to struggle for it, their suffering is intense. This is a steadily increasing nervous contraction, both in the case of the possessed and the possessor, and perfect nervous health is not possible on either side. To begin by respecting the individuality of the baby would put this last abnormal attitude of parent and child out of the question. Curiously enough, there is in some of the worst phases of this parent-child contraction an external appearance of freedom which only enhances the internal slavery. When a man, who has never known what it was in reality to give up a strong will, prides himself upon the freedom he gives to his child, he is entangling himself in the meshes of self-deception, and either depriving another of his own, or ripening him for a good hearty hatred which may at any time mean volcanoes and earthquakes to both.

This forcible resentment of and resistance to the strong will of another is a cause of great nervous suffering, the greater as the expression of such feeling is repressed. Severe illness may easily be the result.

To train a child to gain freedom from the various nervous irritants, one must not only be gaining the same freedom one's self, but must practise meeting the child in the way he is counselled to meet others. One must refuse to be in any way a nervous irritant to the child. In that case quite as much instruction is received as given. A child, too, is doubly sensitive; he not only feels the intrusion on his own individuality, but the irritable or self-willed attitude of another in expressing such intrusion.

Similarly, in keeping a respectful distance, a teacher grows sensitive to the child, and again the help is mutual, with sometimes a balance in favor of the child.

This mistaken, parent-child attitude is often the cause of severe nervous suffering in those whose only relation is that of friendship, when one mind is stronger than the other. Sometimes there is not any real superior strength on the one side; it is simply by the greater gross-ness of the will that the other is overcome. This very grossness blinds one completely to the individuality of a finer strength; the finer individual succumbs because he cannot compete with crowbars, and the parent-child contraction is the disastrous result. To preserve for a child a normal nervous system, one must guide but not limit him. It is a sad sight to see a mother impressing upon a little brain that its owner is a naughty, naughty boy, especially when such impression is increased by the irritability of the mother. One hardly dares to think how many more grooves are made in a child's brain which simply give him contractions to take into mature life with him; how many trivial happenings are made to assume a monstrous form through being misrepresented. It is worth while to think of such dangers, such warping influences, only long enough to avoid them.

A child's imagination is so exquisitely alive, his whole little being is so responsive, that the guidance which can be given him through happy brain-impressions is eminently practicable. To test this responsiveness, and feel it more keenly, just tell a child a dramatic story, and watch his face respond; or even recite a Mother-Goose rhyme with all the expression at your command. The little face changes in rapid succession, as one event after another is related, in a way to put a modern actor to shame. If the response is so quick on the outside, it must be at least equally active within.

One might as well try to make a white rose red by rouging its petals as to mould a child according to one's own idea of what he should be; and as the beauty and delicacy of the rose would be spoiled by the application of the pigment, so is the baby's nervous system twisted and contracted by the limiting force of a grosser will.

Water the rose, put it in the sun, keep the insect enemies away, and then enjoy it for itself. Give the child everything that is consistent with its best growth, but neither force the growth nor limit it; and stand far enough off to see the individuality, to enjoy it and profit by it. Use the child's imagination to calm and strengthen it; give it happy channels for its activity; guide it physically to the rhythm of fresh air, nourishment, and rest; then do not interfere.

If the man never turns to thank you for such guidance, because it all came as a matter of course, a wholesome, powerful nervous system will speak thanks daily with more eloquence than any words could ever express.

XII.

ILLNESS.

AS far as we make circumstances guides and not limitations, they serve us. Otherwise, we serve them, and suffer accordingly. Just in proportion, too, to our allowing circumstances to be limits do we resist them. Such resistance is a nervous strain which disables us physically, and of course puts us more in the clutches of what appears to be our misfortune. The moment we begin to regard every circumstance as an opportunity, the tables are turned on Fate, and we have the upper hand of her.

When we come to think of it, how much common-sense there is in making the best of every "opportunity," and what a lack of sense in chafing at that which we choose to call our limitations! The former way is sure to bring a good result of some sort, be it ever so small; the latter wears upon our nerves, blinds our mental vision, and certainly does not cultivate the spirit of freedom in us.

How absurd it would seem if a wounded man were to expose his wound to unnecessary friction, and then complain that it did not heal! Yet that is what many of us have done at one time or another, when prevented by illness from carrying out our plans in life just as we had arranged. It matters not whether those plans were for ourselves or for others; chafing and fretting at their interruption is just as absurd and quite as sure to delay our recovery. "I know," with tears in our eyes, "I ought not to complain, but it is so hard," To which common-sense may truly answer: "If it is hard, you want to get well, don't you? Then why do you not take every means to get well, instead of indulging first in the very process that will most tend to keep you ill?" Besides this, there is a dogged resistance which remains silent, refuses to complain aloud, and yet holds a state of rigidity that is even worse than the external expression. There are many individual ways of resisting. Each of us knows his own, and knows, too, the futility of it; we do not need to multiply examples.

The patients who resist recovery are quite as numerous as those who keep themselves ill by resisting illness. A person of this sort seems to be fascinated by his own body and its disorders. So far from resisting illness, he may be said to be indulging in it He will talk about himself and his physical state for hours. He will locate each separate disease in a way to surprise the listener by his knowledge of his own anatomy. Not infrequently he will preface a long account of himself by informing you that he has a hearty detestation of talking about himself, and never could understand why people wanted to talk of their diseases. Then in minute detail he will reveal to you his brain-impression of his own case, and look for sympathetic response. These people might recover a hundred times over, and they would never know it, so occupied are they in living their own idea of themselves and in resisting Nature.

When Nature has knocked us down because of disobedience to her laws, we resist her if we attempt at once to rise, or complain of the punishment. When the dear lady would hasten our recovery to the best of her ability, we resist her if we delay progress by dwelling on the punishment or chafing at its necessity.

Nature always tends towards health. It is to prevent further ill-health that she allows us to suffer for our disobedience to her laws. It is to lead us back to health that she is giving the best of her powers, having dealt the deserved punishment. The truest help we can give Nature is not to think of our bodies, well or ill, more than is necessary for their best health.

I knew a woman who was, to all appearances, remarkably well; in fact, her health was her profession. She was supposed to be a Priestess of Health. She talked about and dwelt upon the health of her body until one would have thought there was nothing in the world worth thinking of but a body. She displayed her fine points in the way of health, and enjoyed being questioned with regard to them. This woman was taken ill. She exhibited the same interest, the same pleasure, in talking over and dwelling upon her various forms of illness; in fact, more. She counted her diseases. I am not aware that she ever counted her strong points of health.

This illustration is perhaps clear enough to give a new sense of the necessity for forgetting our bodies. When ill use every necessary remedy; do all that is best to bring renewed health. Having made sure you are doing all you can, forget; don't follow the process. When, as is often the case, pain or other suffering puts forgetting out of the question, use no unnecessary resistance, and forget as soon as the pain is past Don't strengthen the impression by talking about it or telling it over to no purpose. Better forego a little sympathy, and forget the pain sooner.

It is with our nerves that we resist when Nature has punished us. It is nervous strain that we put into a useless attention to and repetition of the details of our illness. Nature wants all this nerve-force to get us well the faster; we can save it for her by not resisting and by a healthy forgetting. By taking an illness as comfortably as possible, and turning our attention to something pleasant outside of ourselves, recovery is made more rapidly.

Many illnesses are accompanied by more or less nervous strain, and its natural control will assist nature and enable medicines to work more quickly. The slowest process of recovery, and that which most needs the relief of a wholesome non-resistance, is when the illness is the result entirely of over-worked nerves. Nature allows herself to be tried to the utmost before she permits nervous prostration. She insists upon being paid in full, principal and interest, before she heals such illness. So severe is she in this case that a patient may appear in every way physically well and strong weeks, nay, months, before he really is so. It was the nerves that broke down last, and the nerves are the last to be restored. It is, however, wonderful to see how much more rapid and certain recovery is if the patient will only separate himself from his nervous system, and refuse all useless strain.

Here are some simple directions which may help nervous patients, if considered in regular order. They can hardly be read too often if the man or woman is in for a long siege; and if simply and steadily obeyed, they will shorten the siege by many days, nay, by many weeks or months, in some cases.

Remember that Nature tends towards health. All you want is nourishment, fresh air, exercise, rest, and patience.

All your worries and anxieties now are tired nerves.

When a worry appears, drop it. If it appears again, drop it again. And so continue to drop it if it appears fifty or a hundred times a day or more.

If you feel like crying, cry; but know that it is the tired nerves that are crying, and don't wonder why you are so foolish,--don't feel ashamed of yourself.

If you cannot sleep, don't care. Get all the rest you can without sleeping. That will bring sleep when it is ready to come, or you are ready to have it.

Don't wonder whether you are going to sleep or not. Go to bed to rest, and let sleep come when it pleases.

Think about everything in Nature. Follow the growing of the trees and flowers. Remember all the beauties in Nature you have ever seen.

Say Mother-Goose rhymes over and over, trying how many you can remember.

Read bright stories for children, and quiet novels, especially Jane Austen's.

Sometimes it helps to work on arithmetic.

Keep aloof from emotions.

Think of other people.

Never think of yourself. Bear in mind that nerves always get well in waves; and if you thought yourself so much better,--almost well, indeed,--and then have a bad time of suffering, don't wonder why it is, or what could have brought it on. Know that it is part of the recovery-process; take it as easily as you can, and then ignore it.

Don't try to do any number of things to get yourself well; don't change doctors any number of times, or take countless medicines. Every doctor knows he cannot hurry your recovery, whatever he may say, and you only retard it by being over-anxious to get strong. Drop every bit of unnecessary muscular tension.

When you walk, feel your feet heavy, as if your shoes were full of lead, and think in your feet.

Be as much like a child as possible. Play with children as one of them, and think with them when you can.

As you begin to recover, find something every day to do for others. Best let it be in the way of house-work, or gardening, or something to do with your hands.

Take care of yourself every day as a matter of course, as you would dress or undress; and be sure that health is coming. Say over and over to yourself: Nourishment, fresh air, exercise, rest, PATIENCE.

When you are well, and resume your former life, if old associations recall the unhappy nervous feelings, know that it is only the associations; pay no attention to the suffering, and work right on. Only be careful to take life very quietly until you are quite used to being well again.

An illness that is merely nervous is an immense opportunity, if one will only realize it as such. It not only makes one more genuinely appreciative of the best health, and the way to keep it, it opens the sympathies and gives a feeling for one's fellow-creatures which, having once found, we cannot prize too highly.

It would seem hard to believe that all must suffer to find a delicate sympathy; it can hardly be so. To be always strong, and at the same time full of warm sympathy, is possible, with more thought. When illness or adverse circumstances bring it, the gate has been opened for us.

If illness is taken as an opportunity to better health, not to more illness, our mental attitude will put complaint out of the question; and as the practice spreads it will as surely decrease the tendency to illness in others as it will shorten its duration in ourselves.

XIII.

SENTIMENT versus SENTIMENTALITY.

FREEDOM from sentimentality opens the way for true sentiment.

An immense amount of time, thought, and nervous force is wasted in sentimentalizing about "being good." With many, the amount of talk about their evils and their desire to overcome them is a thermometer which indicates about five times that amount of thought Neither the talk nor the thought is of assistance in leading to any greater strength or to a more useful life; because the talk is all talk, and the essence of both talk and thought is a selfish, morbid pleasure in dwelling upon one's self. I remember the remark of a young girl who had been several times to prayer-meeting where she heard the same woman say every time that she "longed for the true spirit of religion in her life." With all simplicity, this child said: "If she longs for it, why doesn't she work and find it, instead of coming every week and telling us that she longs?" In all probability the woman returned from every prayer-meeting with the full conviction that, having told her aspirations, she had reached the height desired, and was worthy of all praise.

Prayer-meetings in the old, orthodox sense are not so numerous as they were fifty years ago; but the same morbid love of telling one's own experiences and expressing in words one's own desires for a better life is as common as ever.

Many who would express horror at these public forms of sentimentalizing do not hesitate to indulge in it privately to any extent. Nor do they realize for a moment that it is the same morbid spirit that moves them. It might not be so pernicious a practice if it were not so steadily weakening.

If one has a spark of real desire for better ways of living, sentimentalizing about it is a sure extinguisher if practised for any length of time.

A woman will sometimes pour forth an amount of gush about wishing to be better, broader, nobler, stronger, in a manner that would lead you, for a moment, perhaps, to believe in her sincerity. But when, in the next hour, you see her neglecting little duties that a woman who was really broad, strong, and noble would attend to as a matter of course, and not give a second thought to; when you see that although she must realize that attention to these smaller duties should come first, to open the way to her higher aspirations, she continues to neglect them and continues to aspire,--you are surely right in concluding that she is using up her nervous system in sentimentalizing about a better life; and by that means is doing all in her power to hinder the achievement of it.

It is curious and very sad to see what might be a really strong nature weakening itself steadily with this philosophy and water. Of course it reaches a maudlin state if it continues.

His Satanic Majesty must offer this dose, sweetened with the sugar of self-love, with intense satisfaction. And if we may personify that gentleman for the sake of illustration, what a fine sarcastic smile must dwell upon his countenance as he sees it swallowed and enjoyed, and knows that he did not even have to waste spice as an ingredient! The sugar would have drowned the taste of any spice he could supply.

There is not even the appearance of strength in sentimentalizing.

Besides the sentimentalizing about ourselves in our desire to live a better life, there is the same morbid practice in our love for others; and this is quite as weakening. It contains, of course, no jot of real affection. What wholesome love there is lives in spite of the sentimentalizing, and fortunately is sometimes strong enough on one side or the other to crowd it out and finally exterminate it.

It is curious to notice how often this sham sentiment for others is merely a matter of nerves. As an instance we can take an example, which is quite true, of a woman who fancied herself desperately fond of another, when, much to her surprise, an acute attack of toothache and dentist-fright put the "affection" quite out of her head. In this case the "love" was a nervous irritant, and the toothache a counter-irritant. Of course the sooner such superficial feeling is recognized and shaken off, the nearer we are to real sentiment.

"But," some one will say, "how are we to know what is real and what is not? I would much rather live my life and get more or less unreality than have this everlasting analyzing." There need be no abnormal analyzing; that is as morbid as the other state. Indulge to your heart's content in whatever seems to you real, in what you believe to be wholesome sentiment. But be ready to recognize it as sham at the first hint you get to that effect, and to drop it accordingly.

A perfectly healthy body will shed germs of disease without ever feeling their presence. So a perfectly healthy mind will shed the germs of sentimentality. Few of us are so healthy in mind but that we have to recognize a germ or two and apply a disinfectant before we can reach the freedom that will enable us to shed the germs unconsciously. A good disinfectant is, to refuse to talk of our own feelings or desires or affections, unless for some end which we know may help us to more light and better strength. Talking, however, is mild in its weakening effect compared with thinking. It is better to dribble sham sentiment in words over and over than to think it, and repress the desire to talk. The only clear way is to drop it from our minds the moment it appears; to let go of it as we would loosen our fingers and drop something disagreeable from our hands.

A good amount of exercise and fresh air helps one out of sentimentalizing. This morbid mental habit is often the result of a body ill in some way or another. Frequently it is simply the effect of tired nerves. We help others and ourselves out of it more rapidly by not mentioning the sentimentalizing habit, but by taking some immediate means towards rest, fresh air, vigorous exercise, and better nourishment.

Mistakes are often made and ourselves or others kept an unnecessary length of time in mental suffering because we fail to attribute a morbid mental state to its physical cause. We blame ourselves or others for behavior that we call wicked or silly, and increase the suffering, when all that is required is a little thoughtful care of the body to cause the silly wickedness to disappear entirely.

We are supposed to be indulging in sickly sentiment when we are really suffering from sickly nerves. An open sympathy will detect this mistake very soon, and save intense suffering by an early remedy.

Sentiment is as strengthening as sentimentality is weakening. It is as strong, as clear, and as fine in flavor as the other is sickly sweet. No one who has tasted the wholesome vigor of the one could ever care again for the weakening sweetness of the other, however much he might have to suffer in getting rid of it. True sentiment seeks us; we do not seek it. It not only seeks us, it possesses us, and runs in our blood like the new life which comes from fresh air on top of a mountain. With that true sentiment we can feel a desire to know better things and to live them. We can feel a hearty love for others; and a love that is, in its essence, the strongest of all human loves. We can give and receive a healthy sympathy which we could never have known otherwise. We can enjoy talking about ourselves and about" being good," because every word we say will be spontaneous and direct, with more thought of law than of self. This true sentiment seeks and finds us as we recognize the sham and shake it off, and as we refuse to dwell upon our actions and thoughts in the past or to look back at all except when it is a necessity to gain a better result.

We are like Orpheus, and true sentiment is our Eurydice with her touch on our shoulder; the spirits that follow are the sham-sentiments, the temptations to look back and pose. The music of our lyre is the love and thought we bring to our every-day life. Let us keep steadily on with the music, and lead our Eurydice right through Hades until we have her safely over the Lethe, and we know sentimentality only as a name.

XIV.

PROBLEMS.

THERE are very few persons who have not I had the experience of giving up a problem in mathematics late in the evening, and waking in the morning with the solution clear in their minds. That has been the experience of many, too, in real-life problems. If it were more common, a great amount of nervous strain might be saved.

There are big problems and little, real and imaginary; and some that are merely tired nerves. In problems, the useless nervous element often plays a large part. If the "problems" were dropped out of mind with sufferers from nervous prostration, their progress towards renewed health might be just twice as rapid. If they were met normally, many nervous men and women might be entirely saved from even a bowing acquaintance with nervous prostration. It is not a difficult matter, that of meeting a problem normally,-- simply let it solve itself. In nine cases out of ten, if we leave it alone and live as if it were not, it will solve itself. It is at first a matter of continual surprise to see how surely this self-solution is the result of a wholesome ignoring both of little problems and big ones.

In the tenth case, where the problem must be faced at once, to face it and decide to the best of our ability is, of course, the only thing to do. But having decided, be sure that it ceases to be a problem. If we have made a mistake, it is simply a circumstance to guide us for similar problems to come.

All this is obvious; we know it, and have probably said it to ourselves dozens of times. If we are sufferers from nervous problems, we may have said it dozens upon dozens of times. The trouble is that we have said it and not acted upon it. When a problem will persist in worrying us, in pulling and dragging upon our nerves, an invitation to continue the worrying until it has worked itself out is a great help towards its solution or disappearance.

I remember once hearing a bright woman say that when there was anything difficult to decide in her life she stepped aside and let the opposing elements fight it out within her. Presumably she herself threw in a little help on one side or the other which really decided the battle. But the help was given from a clear standpoint, not from a brain entirely befogged in the thick of the fight

Whatever form problems may take, however important they may seem, when they attack tired nerves they must be let alone. A good way is to go out into the open air and so identify one's self with Nature that one is drawn away in spite of one's self. A big wind will sometimes blow a brain clear of nervous problems in a very little while if we let it have its will. Another way out is to interest one's self in some game or other amusement, or to get a healthy interest in other people's affairs, and help where we can.

Each individual can find his own favorite escape. Of course we should never shirk a problem that must be decided, but let us always wait a reasonable time for it to decide itself first. The solving that is done for us is invariably better and clearer than any we could do for ourselves.

It will be curious, too, to see how many apparently serious problems, relieved of the importance given them by a strained nervous system, are recognized to be nothing at all. They fairly dissolve themselves and disappear.

XV.

SUMMARY.

THE line has not been clearly drawn, either in general or by individuals, between true civilization and the various perversions of the civilizing process. This is mainly because we do not fairly face the fact that the process of civilization is entirely according to Nature, and that the perversions which purport to be a direct outcome of civilization are, in point of fact, contradictions or artificialities which are simply a going-over into barbarism, just as too far east is west.

If you suggest "Nature" in habits and customs to most men nowadays, they at once interpret you to mean "beastly," although they would never use the word.

It is natural to a beast to be beastly: he could not be anything else; and the true order of his life as a beast is to be respected. It is natural to a man to govern himself, as he possesses the power of distinguishing and choosing, With all the senses and passions much keener, and in their possibilities many degrees finer, than the beasts, he has this governing power, which makes his whole nervous system his servant just in so far as through this servant he loyally obeys his own natural laws. A man in building a bridge could never complain when he recognized that it was his obedience to the laws of mechanics which enabled him to build the bridge, and that he never could have arbitrarily arranged laws that would make the bridge stand. In the same way, one who has come to even a slight recognition of the laws that enable him to be naturally civilized and not barbarously so, steadily gains, not only a realization of the absolute futility of resisting the laws, but a growing respect and affection for them.

It is this sham civilization, this selfish refinement of barbarous propensities, this clashing of nervous systems instead of the clashing of weapons, which has been largely, if not entirely, the cause of such a variety and extent of nervous trouble throughout the so-called civilized world. It is not confined to nervous prostration; if there is a defective spot organically, an inherited tendency to weakness, the nervous irritation is almost certain to concentrate upon it instead of developing into a general nervous break-down.

With regard to a cure for all this, no superficial remedy, such as resting and feeding, is going to prove of lasting benefit; any more than a healing salve will suffice to do away with a blood disease which manifests itself by sores on the surface of the skin. No physician would for a moment inveigle himself into the belief that the use of external means alone would cure a skin disease that was caused by some internal disorder. Such skin irritation may be easily cured by the right remedy, whereas an external salve would only be a means of repression, and would result in much greater trouble subsequently.

Imagine a man superficially cured of an illness, and then exposed while yet barely convalescent to influences which produce a relapse. That is what is done in many cases when a patient is rested, and fattened like a prize pig, and then sent home into all the old conditions, with nothing to help him to elude them but a well-fed, well-rested body. That, undeniably, means a great deal for a short period; but the old conditions discover the scars of old wounds, and the process of reopening is merely a matter of time. From all sides complaints are heard of the disastrous results of civilization; while with even a slight recognition of the fact that the trouble was caused by the rudiments of barbarism, and that the higher civilization is the life which is most truly natural, remedies for our nervous disorders would be more easily found.

It is the perversions of the natural process of civilization that do the harm; just as with so-called domesticated flowers there arise coarse abnormal growths, and even diseases, which the wholesome, delicate organism of a wild flower makes impossible.

The trouble is that we do not know our own best powers at all; the way is stopped so effectually by this persistent nervous irritation. With all its superficiality, it is enough to impede the way to the clear, nervous strength which is certainly our inheritance.

After all, what has been said in the foregoing chapters is simply illustrative of a prevalent mental skin-disorder.

If the whole world were suffering from a physical cutaneous irritation, the minds of individuals would be so concentrated on their sensations that no one could know of various wonderful powers in his own body which are now taken as a matter of course. There would be self-consciousness in every physical action, because it must come through, and in spite of, external irritation. Just in so far as each individual one of us found and used the right remedy for our skin-trouble should we be free to discover physical powers that were unknown to our fellow-sufferers, and free to help them to a similar remedy when they were willing to be helped.

This mental skin-disorder is far more irritating and more destructive, and not only leads to, but actually is, in all its forms, a sort of self-consciousness through which we work with real difficulty.

To discover its shallowness and the simplicity of its cure is a boon we can hardly realize until, by steady application, we have found the relief. The discovery and cure do not lead to a millennium any more than the cure of any skin disease guarantees permanent health. For deeper personal troubles there are other remedies. Each will recognize and find his own; but freedom, through and through, can never be found, or even looked for clearly, while the irritation from the skin disease is withdrawing our attention.

"But, friends, Truth is within ourselves: it takes no rise From outward things; whatever you may believe, There is an inmost centre in us all Where truth abides in fulness; and around, Wall upon wall, the gross flesh hems it in, This perfect clear perception which is truth. A baffling and perverting carnal mesh Blinds it, and makes all error; and TO KNOW Rather consists in opening out a way Whence the imprisoned splendor may escape, Than in effecting entry for a light Supposed to be without."

Browning's "baffling and perverting carnal mesh" might be truly interpreted as a nervous tangle which is nothing at all except as we make it with our own perverted sight.

To help us to move a little distance from the phantom tangle, that it may disappear before our eyes, has been the aim of this book. So by curing our mental skin-disease as a matter of course, and then forgetting that it ever existed, we may come to real life. This no one can find for another, but each has within himself the way.

THE END.